D1049080

HEALTHY YOU
HEALTHY BABY

A mother's guide to gestational diabetes

By the Doctor's Dietitian
Susan B. Dopart, MS, RD, CDE

To our daughter Grace Anne.
You could not be a part of our lives,
but you are my little angel who helps me
support bringing healthy babies into this world.

Edition 1, First Printing: April 2012

Copyright @ 2012 Susan B. Dopart

G SGJ Publishing
Santa Monica, California

Publisher's Cataloging-In-Publication Data
(Prepared by The Donohue Group, Inc.)

Dopart, Susan B.

   Healthy you, healthy baby : a mother's guide to gestational diabetes / by Susan B. Dopart. -- [1st ed.].

   p. : ill., charts ; cm.

   "By the Doctor's Dietitian."
Includes bibliographical references and index.
ISBN: 978-0-615-51825-1

   1. Diabetes in pregnancy--Popular works. 2. Pregnancy--Nutritional aspects--Popular works. 3. Pregnant women--Health and hygiene--Guidebooks. I. Title.

RG580.D5 D67 2012
618.364/6

A Note to Readers

The information in this book is not intended or implied to be a substitute for professional medical advice, diagnosis or treatment. All content in these pages -- including text, charts, illustrations, graphics and photographs -- is for general information purposes only.

You are encouraged to confirm any information obtained from or through this book with other sources, and to review all information regarding any medical condition or treatment with your physician or healthcare professional.

Never disregard professional medical advice, forego or delay seeking medical treatment because of something you have read in this book.

Table of Contents

How did I get here and what should I do now
that I have GDM?

A. Insulin resistance
B. Carbohydrates
C. Protein
D. Fat
E. Balancing your meals

A. Goals to achieve – normal vs. high sugars
B. Glucometers
C. Factors affecting glucose levels
   – food, exercise, sleep and stress
D. Interpreting your results

Foreword

Dear reader,

Gestational diabetes mellitus (GDM) has become one of the major medical complications among pregnant women. On average, about one out of five American women develop gestational diabetes. However, the rates may be doubled among Asian or Hispanic women, obese women, or among women with high weight gains, especially in the early weeks of pregnancy.

Learning how to prevent GDM, or how to manage the disease if you have already been diagnosed, is the most important step you can take.

GDM has been treated by diet for more than 125 years. Today, diet is the first choice for managing blood glucose levels. Many women control their blood glucose levels by eating healthy foods so they do not need any medications. Registered dietitian Susan B. Dopart, one of my former students at UC Berkeley, has a personal interest in diabetes as it runs in her family. She has lived this diet and is sharing her own experiences with you.

As you read through the book, you will quickly learn how to adjust your usual pattern of eating to a more healthy one by adding some new foods and eliminating others. Also, your entire family can eat just like you, and there is no need to change your diet after the baby is born. Sometimes women who have GDM develop diabetes after their pregnancies. The diet described in this book will reduce your risk of diabetes throughout your life.

It is not easy to change your eating habits, and you don't have to do it all at once.

You might start by focusing on one aspect of your diet such as fruits and vegetables one week and then another the next week. Knowing why these changes benefit your health and that of your baby makes it a lot easier to shift your diet.

Remember, you are not alone in managing your health. You have a team of healthcare providers to help you. But, you are the head of your healthcare team, and you are the one who will benefit by making positive changes in your diet.

Finally, don't forget to enjoy your pregnancy. With this book in hand, you have started a journey of improving your health and that of your entire family. As you shift to more healthy foods, congratulate yourself for a job well done.

Janet C. King, PhD
Senior Scientist, Children's Hospital Oakland
Research Institute Professor, UC Berkeley and UC Davis

Acknowledgements

This book was born out of my passion for helping women create healthy lifestyles they can pass on to future generations. There were many who helped bring this book to life.

I want to thank my colleagues who gave their time in editing, feedback and encouragement: Ruth Garland, RN, CDE; Erika Demonsant, RD; and Pamela Lee, MPH, RD, CDE.

Besides encouragement and editing, Deborah Norman-Lesin, RN, BSN, CDE, was an inspiration for this book and supported me throughout the entire process.

To Janet King, PhD, for her important foreword for this book, for starting me on the road to understanding the biochemistry of nutrition, and never wavering on the science of food.

Many thanks to Deborah Frank, CNM, for her encouragement, support and endorsement for this book and the nurturing care she gives in helping to bring healthy babies into the world.

To Michelle Williams, ScD, for her support in endorsing this book and all the scientific research she provides to ensure women with GDM get the best care they need as a result of her research.

Great appreciation to Sheryl Ross, MD, for her encouragement and for trusting me with the care of her GDM patients. I value our partnership and shared purpose to create an environment for healthy babies.

Special thanks to the women who contributed their stories to help other women with GDM: Jessica, Leslie, Wendy and Andie.

To Joni Donnella for contributing her time and beautiful bump for the front cover. Special thanks to Jonathan Davino, Josh Sanseri, Sam Nazarian, Dante Dauz and Andrew Bick for help with photography and the book cover. Special thanks to Rachel Morrison, Ramona Trent Photography and JEM Photography for contributing some beautiful pictures.

Special thanks to Debra Main for her amazing support, wisdom and assistance with design, editing and clarity with direction for this book.

I want to thank my parents, Evangeline and Joseph Dopart, for editing this book and providing support for all my endeavors.

To Jessica Liu Brookshire for her incredible talent for design. She foresaw my design for this book before I even conveyed it to her. With her talent, the pages of this book came to life.

I want to especially extend gratitude to my editor, Catherine Wire Roberts, for her dedication to my writing, her beautiful spirit and innovative style. She is truly the Renaissance woman in every respect. Despite having a demanding day job and family commitments, she always makes time for my projects and books. There are really no words to express my appreciation to her.

And lastly, I thank my partner in life, Jeffrey Batchelor, for his encouragement in writing this book and his unwavering assistance with editing, photography and support. Jeffrey had the vision of me writing this book before I ever knew it, and he encouraged me through every step of the process.

Susan B. Dopart, MS, RD, CDE

What should I do now that I have Gestational Diabetes?

If you are holding this guide in your hands, you probably have more questions than answers right now:

> *Is my baby going to be okay?*
> *Was it something I was eating?*
> *Did I do something wrong?*

Gestational diabetes (GDM) is a complex endocrinology disorder caused by multiple factors. It may be in your genes, your weight prior to pregnancy, what you ate, how active you are, etc. However, trying to solve this mystery is not going to help you now and may even hinder you from getting the information and treatment you need. It is more important to focus on **WHAT TO DO** next to keep you and your baby healthy for the remainder of your pregnancy.

My Approach

Diabetes runs strong in my genes. Although I have not had diabetes, I do everything possible to avoid getting it. I became a dietitian to help others avoid the occurrence and consequences of diabetes. I attend numerous diabetes conferences to make sure I am up-to-date on medical and nutritional information that will help me assist my patients.

With the goal of the best possible outcome for you and your baby, this book contains current, cutting-edge information on GDM from leading physicians and researchers from all over the world.

Most importantly, I will tell you exactly what you need to do to keep your blood sugars balanced and normal. With blood glucose testing, food combinations and exercise, I hope to help you eliminate your need for medications.

Current research shows that women with GDM who are successfully treated have outcomes equal to women without GDM. How's that for some good news? In addition, 70 percent of women with GDM can develop type two diabetes within 10 years if their diets or lifestyles remain unchanged. Therefore, a lifestyle change now is an opportunity to lower your risk of future diabetes - a blessing in disguise!

As you go through this book, you will hear from women with GDM. I hope their stories will encourage you and help you realize that taking steps to help your baby will also help your own future health. Changing your lifestyle can influence the health of future generations of women and children in your own lineage.

So, put aside your worries, and together we will embark on a journey to better health, a successful pregnancy and a healthy baby.

Susan B. Dopart, MS, RD, CDE

The GDM Diet

Taking the best care of your child's future health starts with what happens in the womb. What you consume during pregnancy can determine whether your child:

- Is born too small or large *(called small for gestation or large for gestation)*
- Starts off with a predisposition toward normal weight versus obesity
- Is predisposed to having diabetes, heart disease or cancer
- Has a high cholesterol or triglyceride level at birth leading to fatty liver

These realities show how self-care through diet and exercise is of the utmost importance.

A baby is programmed in the womb with a certain set of genes or DNA, but how he or she responds to that DNA can be influenced by your diet and level of self care.

Epigenetics is a term scientists use to describe their point of view that genes are controlled beyond what is encoded in DNA. As a mother, you have a powerful impact on the future health of your child – both a wonderful and a daunting responsibility. You can't change your genes, but you can control your diet.

The diet for GDM is a healthy way of eating and differs slightly from the diet for other types of diabetes. The goal of the GDM diet is to keep blood glucose levels normalized during pregnancy. Hormones during pregnancy can cause changes in your blood sugars, thereby needing adjustments in the diet.

No doubt you've heard of carbohydrate, protein and fat. These three macronutrients and how they are combined determine whether your blood glucose levels will be normal or elevated. To better understand what happens to your body, let's first talk about **insulin resistance** – the underlying reason for GDM.

Understanding Insulin Resistance

Normally insulin, a hormone released from the pancreas, enables cells to remove glucose (sugar) from the bloodstream to be used as energy (see diagram on page 16). Approximately one-third of the population inherits a trait whereby their cells respond improperly to insulin. This results in higher circulating levels of blood glucose, which causes the pancreas to release ever-increasing amounts of insulin in an attempt to normalize blood glucose levels. This can eventually lead to diabetes.

Simply put, insulin is the key that unlocks the cell for sugar to get in, which in turn, enables your body to use the food you consume. However, somewhere along the line, the key either gets stuck or has difficulty getting into the lock. Or, if it does get in, it cannot turn the lock. Therefore, it was given the term "resistant." If your body develops a resistance to insulin, you are not able to utilize the food you take in. This can increase your fatigue and cravings for ever-greater amounts of carbohydrate, which compounds the problem.

This resistance sets up a cascade of reactions in the body that are not in your favor. It is as if the sugar is outside the cell knocking to get in. When it cannot get in, your body keeps craving more carbohydrate. Sort of like when you eat one slice of bread then find yourself wanting the whole loaf.

Insulin Resistance & Pregnancy

Since pregnancy is a state of insulin resistance, many women are susceptible to blood glucose changes. Scientifically, *gestational diabetes mellitus* is defined as carbohydrate intolerance of variable severity with onset of first recognition during pregnancy. [1]

As you get farther along in your pregnancy, the placenta grows, which increases the level of insulin resistance with each week. At about 20-24 weeks gestation, the hormones the placenta makes (estrogen, cortisol, progesterone, and human placental lactogen) begin to partially block the action of insulin. The body responds by making more insulin, but sometimes it is not enough, and the result is gestational diabetes.

Women who already have adult onset, or type two diabetes, can have higher levels of insulin resistance with resulting higher blood glucose levels. They may need to alter their diets at this point in the pregnancy or increase their oral medications or insulin dosages due to these metabolic changes.

How can we control or quiet insulin resistance to help with normalizing your blood glucose levels? Let's start with the balance of what you are eating.

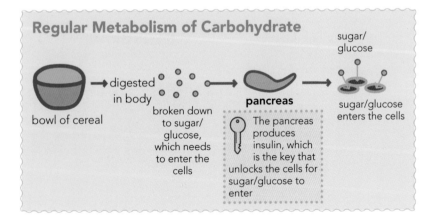

Regular Metabolism of Carbohydrate

sugar/glucose

bowl of cereal → digested in body → broken down to sugar/glucose, which needs to enter the cells

pancreas → The pancreas produces insulin, which is the key that unlocks the cells for sugar/glucose to enter

sugar/glucose enters the cells

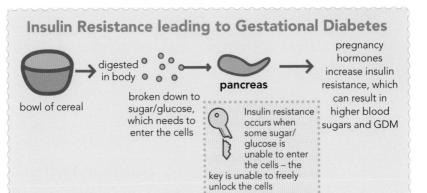

Insulin Resistance leading to Gestational Diabetes

bowl of cereal

digested in body

broken down to sugar/glucose, which needs to enter the cells

pancreas

Insulin resistance occurs when some sugar/glucose is unable to enter the cells – the key is unable to freely unlock the cells

pregnancy hormones increase insulin resistance, which can result in higher blood sugars and GDM

Carbohydrate: Good Carbs vs. Bad Carbs

Understanding the difference between carbohydrates is essential to learning how to eat healthfully. If you are eating food in its purest form – i.e. food which is not processed - then it is likely that you are eating a healthy form of carbohydrate.

Examples of foods that contain healthy forms of carbohydrates include:

- fruits and vegetables
- low-fat plain dairy products
- nuts and seeds
- whole grains such as brown rice, quinoa and buckwheat
- beans/legumes

Examples of foods that contain processed and low-fiber carbo-hydrates:

- pasta, potatoes, white rice
- white bread, bagels, English muffins and muffins
- crackers, chips, pretzels
- most breakfast cereals
- pancakes and waffles
- ready-made desserts

Unfortunately, our culture has accepted the idea that eating grains means consuming bread, rice pasta and potatoes in any form. These foods are low in fiber and nutrients and are essentially "filler foods."

How Many Slices?

One useful way to understand carbohydrate equivalents is to compare them to a slice of bread (any type), which contains approximately 15 grams of carbohydrate. This is what the American Diabetes Association uses as one serving of carbohydrate.

Therefore, just as one serving of carbohydrate equals 15 grams, two servings equals 30 grams and so forth. Knowing this, you can look at any label and see how many servings or slices of bread's worth of carbohydrate you are consuming.

For example, this label is for a 4-oz plain bagel. It contains 61 grams of total carbohydrate, which is equal to four slices of bread. Few people would eat four slices of bread at breakfast, but many could easily eat this bagel.

Nutrition Facts

Serving Size (113g)
Servings Per Container

Amount Per Serving

Calories 310   Calories from Fat 15

% Daily Value*

Total Fat 2g	**3%**
Saturated Fat 0g	**0%**
Trans Fat --g	
Cholesterol 0mg	**0%**
Sodium 610mg	**25%**
Total Carbohydrate 61g	**20%**
Dietary Fiber 3g	**10%**
Sugars --g	
Protein 12g	

Vitamin A 0%	Vitamin C 0%
Calcium 2%	Iron 8%

*Percent Daily Values are based on a 2,000 calorie diet. Your daily values may be higher or lower depending on your calorie needs:

	Calories:	2,000	2,500
Total Fat	Less than	65g	80g
Saturated Fat	Less than	20g	25g
Cholesterol	Less than	300mg	300mg
Sodium	Less than	2,400mg	2,400mg
Total Carbohydrate		300g	375g
Dietary Fiber		25g	30g

Calories per gram:
Fat 9 • Carbohydrate 4 • Protein 4

Many times we are unaware that we are taking in excessive carbohydrates. Reading labels is a great tool for knowing how many carbohydrates you are consuming.

Unmask Hidden Sugars

In addition to reading the label for total amounts of carbohy-drate, it may be necessary to check the label for ingredients or names that indicate components for sugars or starches – such as sucrose, dextrose, fructose, maltose, glucose, mannitol, sorbitol, molasses, monosaccharides, polysaccharides, maple syrup, date sugar, brown sugar, raw sugar, turbinado sugar, high fructose corn syrup, brown rice syrup or agave.

Hidden sources of sugar can drive up your glucose readings, so pay attention to ingredients!

Types of Carbohydrates – Nature Knows Best

Carbohydrate coming from sources in their natural state do not affect the blood sugar as dramatically as those that have been altered by man in some way. For example, carbohydrates coming from vegetables, fruits, nuts/seeds, avocado, etc. do not affect the blood sugars in the same way as carbohydrates coming from starches such as white rice, pasta and cereals.

Some natural starches, like potatoes, can also dramatically raise your glucose levels. Testing your blood sugars 1-2 hours after the first bite of a meal shows how particular foods affect your levels, so testing is essential. Various starches or types of carbohydrates can raise one individual's blood glucose level more than another.

Women with GDM may be more sensitive to the combination of carbohydrates coming from fruit (fructose) and milk (lactose). These sugars can have the greatest impact at *breakfast.* Some women consuming one or both of these sugars can experience higher glucose levels than just having one at a time. Some guidelines indicate not having either fructose or lactose at breakfast.

Breakfast sets the tone for the rest of the day. Since you are most insulin resistant in the morning, figuring out how much and what type of carbohydrates your body handles will ultimately be determined by your glucose readings. (Continued on page 22)

Carbohydrate Equivalents

Carbohydrate-containing foods are: fruits, vegetables, dairy products, nuts, seeds, whole grains, beans, and legumes. This list includes many foods that are classically counted as being one carbohydrate serving.

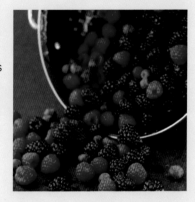

A healthy servings of carbohydrate (equal to about 15 grams of carbohydrate) – include these foods in your diet:

½ cup of fresh fruit (citrus, melon, grapes, cherries, peaches, plums)

1 cup of berries (blueberries, strawberries, raspberries)

1 medium fruit (apple, orange, peach, etc.)

½ medium banana

½ large fruit (grapefruit, papaya, large apple)

2 cups of non-starchy vegetables (broccoli, cauliflower, zucchini)

10 cups of lettuce or mixed greens (romaine, butter, spinach)

½ cup of starchy vegetables (peas, beans, corn)

½ cup of whole grains (brown rice, quinoa and buckwheat)

½ cup of beans (kidney, pinto, garbanzo, navy)

½ cup of yams, sweet potatoes and potatoes

1 medium slice of whole wheat bread

½ cup of cooked steel-cut oats

1 cup of one percent milk

1 cup of plain yogurt

Processed forms of carbohydrate (equal to about 15 grams of carbohydrate) – Limit these foods:

1 medium slice of white bread

¼ of a bagel

1 ounce of unsweetened cereal

1 corn or whole wheat tortilla

¾ cup of cooked cereal

½ cup of cooked pasta or white rice

3-4 small-to medium-sized crackers

1 cup of noodle-or rice-based soup

1 crust of a medium slice of pizza

Other foods that contain approximately 15 grams of carbohydrate – Limit or avoid these foods:

½ cup of fruit juice (orange, apple, grape)

2 small cookies

1 small slice of unfrosted cake

½ cup of regular ice cream

⅓ cup nonfat frozen yogurt

1 dollar-size pancake

1 tablespoon of maple syrup, honey, jelly/jam

Varying amounts of breakfast cereals and desserts

1 ounce of savory snack foods (potato chips, pretzels, etc.)

A Quick Check After Breakfast

Checking your blood glucose levels after breakfast will show you whether you are sensitive to either fructose or lactose being consumed at the same time or if you are sensitive to having either fruit (fructose) or milk (lactose) at breakfast.

Your total grams of carbohydrate are divided among all your meals and snacks according to your blood glucose values. Current guidelines for women with GDM recommend a minimum of 175 grams of total carbohydrates per day with absolute minimum of 150 grams. However, additional grams may be needed if ketones are present.

Ketones are produced when there is an insufficient amount of insulin necessary to allow glucose or sugar to get into your cells. The body uses fat or muscle for energy instead of the food you are eating.

Doing a simple urine test will determine whether your body is making ketones. Ketone sticks can be purchased at most pharmacies without a prescription. If the test is negative, no further action is necessary. However, if ketones are present, you will need to add more carbohydrate to your diet.

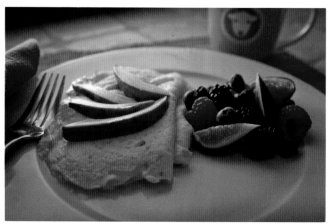

Example of a healthy GDM breakfast

Protein

A good motto is to think of protein as your friend. Having protein at each meal and at snack time blunts the spike in your blood glucose that results from carbohydrate alone. The resulting insulin levels from the combination of protein and carbohydrate help to create an even keel in your body and blood glucose levels.

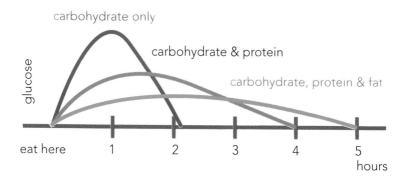

Meal balance
If you eat a high-carbohydrate, low-protein breakfast, insulin levels can increase sharply, causing your blood sugar to crash within 2 - 2½ hours, stimulating hunger. If you eat a balance of protein, healthy fat, and moderate amounts of carbohydrate, insulin levels will rise more moderately, causing your blood sugars and appetite to be at a more even keel.

Recent studies have demonstrated that adequate protein is essential during pregnancy for beta cell production. **Beta cells** are contained in the pancreas and produce the insulin to help nutrients get into the cells of your body. When a mother is consuming a low level of protein, it blocks the cells from becoming beta cells, which affects her body's ability to make enough insulin. [2]

Protein is responsible not only for balancing your blood sugars, but also for keeping your pancreas efficient. Protein is essential during pregnancy for:

- Growth and repair of every cell in your body and your baby's body
- Building strong muscles and bones
- Making antibodies that play a role in immunity
- Production of red and white blood cells
- Feeling satiated and full after a meal

Examples of high-protein foods:

- meat, poultry, fish
- hard cheeses, cottage or ricotta cheese
- plain yogurt, milk
- eggs
- nuts/seeds and nut butters
- beans and legumes
- soybeans, tofu, and tempeh

Having adequate protein throughout the day is essential to achieving blood glucose balance, keeping satisfied and having the energy you need. Shortchanging yourself on protein can result in low or high blood sugars, constant carbohydrate cravings, and unhealthy levels of hunger and fatigue.

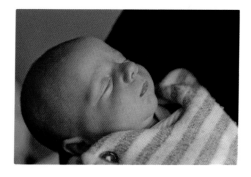

Protein Equivalents

A serving of protein is 7-8 grams on a label. Normally we consume about 3-6 servings of protein per meal, or about 21-48 grams of protein. A serving of protein is equal to:

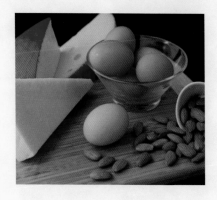

1 ounce of hard cheese (Cheddar, Swiss, Monterey Jack, Havarti, mozzarella or other hard cheeses)

¼ cup of low-fat cottage cheese

¼ cup of part-skim ricotta cheese

2 tablespoons of parmesan cheese

1½ ounces of feta or goat cheese

1 cup of 1% milk

1 cup of plain yogurt

1 egg

2 egg whites

1 ounce of lean beef, lamb, pork, poultry, or fish

1½ ounces of shellfish (shrimp, crab, lobster)

¼ cup of canned tuna or salmon

¼ cup of natto (fermented soybeans)

¼ cup of tempeh

4 ounces of tofu or about ½ cup*

¼ cup of soybeans (edamame)*

2 tablespoons of raw nuts or seeds

2 tablespoons of natural peanut or other nut butters such as cashew or almond

½ cup of beans (kidney, pinto, garbanzo, navy)

*These soy products contain phytic acid which can lower absorption of iron, zinc, calcium and magnesium

Fat

Fat is essential in many ways during pregnancy and can affect many aspects of your baby's development. Fat is the structure of cells in the body, but more importantly, it influences the structure of your child's brain. Eating healthy sources of fat is critical.

Fat is so important that without it we would not be alive. Here are the reasons why:

- It supplies essential fatty acids the body cannot manufacture that are needed for healthy skin, hair and brain development in utero
- Fats are critical in the structure and function of all cells and the nervous system
- Fat is needed for proper digestion and absorption of fat-soluble vitamins (A, E, D, and K)
- Sixty percent of the dry weight of the brain is fat, and healthy neurons contain a type of fat known as DHA

Since different types of fat exist, here is a quick synopsis of what they are and how they work since they are an important part of pregnancy.

Saturated fat was once thought to be the villain, and many healthcare professionals recommended avoiding all sources of saturated fat. We now know that having some saturated fat will not break your health bank and some types of saturated fat are a healthy part of pregnancy. Two sources of healthy saturated fats are organic butter and extra-virgin, organic coconut oil. Coconut oil contains a type of oil called lauric acid that is only found here and in mother's breast milk. Lauric acid is a powerful immune stimulant and may help in preventing sickness.

Polyunsaturated fat is divided into different categories – omega-3 fats and omega-6 fats – and it is important to under-stand the difference between them.

Monounsaturated fat is associated with a lowered risk of heart disease since it can lower the HDL or good cholesterol. Examples of monounsaturated fat are avocados, nuts/seeds and olive oil and are an important part of a healthy diet.

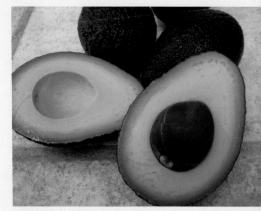

Avocados: packed with healthy monounsaturated fats

Fat Equivalents

One serving of fat is approximately equal to 5 grams of fat on a label. A reasonable amount of fat is 1-3 servings per meal. Approximately 5 grams of fat is equal to:

1 teaspoon of oil (olive preferred)

1 teaspoon of butter

1 tablespoon of salad dressing

1 tablespoon of cream cheese

1 tablespoon of sour cream

1 tablespoon of guacamole

⅓ of a medium avocado

Omega-6 fats are plentiful in the diet, so it is not necessary to focus on getting more. In fact, it may be necessary to lower your intake of omega-6 fats since they are thought to increase inflammation in the body. Since diabetes is thought to be low-grade inflammation, limiting intake of omega-6 fats can be helpful in lowering your blood glucose levels.

Omega-6 fats are present in oils such as soybean, corn, vegetable, cottonseed and safflower. These oils are the ones we frequently see in processed, packaged foods because they are inexpensive and have longer shelf lives.

If you are consuming products from corn-fed animals (versus grass-fed like our ancestors the cavemen) you are receiving omega-6 fats.

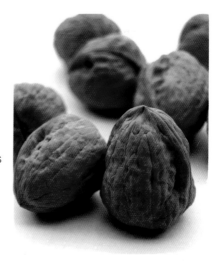

Increasing **omega-3 fats** during pregnancy may be one of the most important steps in helping your blood

Walnuts: packed with monounsaturated and omega-3 fatty acids

sugars. Omega-3 fats can reduce the chances of your child being overweight at birth, having a high cholesterol level or internal inflammation – all of which set the stage for their future health. Studies show higher levels of omega-3 fats can lower a mother's triglyceride levels by 10 percent, which can decrease the chance of an overweight infant.[3] Triglycerides are the storage form of fat in the blood and are associated with insulin resistance.

Boost Your Omega-3 Fats

Next, let's look at the kinds of omega-3 fats that exist and how can you incorporate them into your diet. Here are the big three:

- alpha-linolenic acid (ALA)
- eicosapentaenoic acid (EPA)
- docosahexaenoic acid (DHA)

ALA is called an *essential fatty acid* because the body cannot manufacture it on its own, and therefore you have to ingest the right foods to get it. The highest concentration of ALA is found in flaxseed, but it can also be found in green leafy vegetables and flaxseed oil. If you include one tablespoon of ground flax-seed in your diet per day, it will provide all your ALA needs.

Rich sources of EPA and DHA are fatty fish and fish oils. The American Heart Association recommends eating fatty fish at least twice a week to have a diet high in EPA and DHA. Salmon has approximately 300 mg. of DHA per ounce. Halibut contains approximately 80 mg. of DHA per ounce. Therefore, if you had a 3-ounce piece of either of these fish, you would be receiving 900 and 240 mg. respectively.

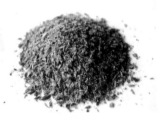

Ground flax seeds

Even if you eat fish, taking a fish oil supplement, either in oil or capsule form, ensures you are receiving this essential fat. Omega-3 fats feed your brain and that of your baby. In order for your body to work efficiently, your brain needs to be properly fed or saturated with enough good fat. An average, well-nourished brain should have about 20 grams of DHA at all times, or about 20 fish oil capsules. If you consume the recommended amount of fish oil per day (see below) your brain will contain adequate DHA. Many health professionals now believe it is essential to feed the body from the brain down!

In prehistoric times, cavemen ate a Paleolithic diet consisting of large amounts of wild fish or beef raised on grass (versus corn or grains) and therefore, ate larger amounts of DHA than the standard American diet, which provides barely 100 mg. of DHA per day.

In the past, many people have been turned off by the taste of fish oil, but it has become more user friendly in the last year. There is lemon-flavored fish oil and other various flavors of fish oil that taste good. The amazing thing about fish oil is that you can add it to a salad dressing without compromising the flavor. If you can't stomach the fish oil, many companies make fish oil capsules. Look at the back of the label for DHA and EPA content. The recommended amount is a minimum of 500-1000 mg. **each** of DHA and EPA. Many times the outside of the bottle states "1000 mg. of omega-3 fats," but does not give the breakdown for EPA and DHA. Therefore, it is necessary to read the label for the exact amounts.

What to look for on a label:

- EPA: 500-1000 mg.
- DHA: 500-1000 mg.

The combination of taking one tablespoon of ground flaxseed and at least 500 mg. each of DHA and EPA via fish oil ensures you are receiving adequate omega fats to help not only your blood sugars, but assist with brain development of your child.

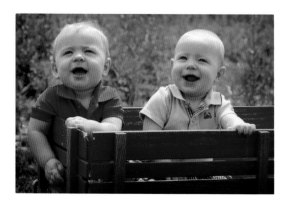

Fish and Pregnancy

Advocating the consumption of fish and fish oil may seem at odds with what you might have heard about the dangers of eating fish while pregnant, so I'll explain. Many fish are grown in mercury-rich waters and are unhealthy to consume. Wild fish (as opposed to farmed fish) contain far less mercury and provide the omega-3 fatty acids that are essential to health. Some farmed fish, including farmed salmon, can contain PCBs (polychlorinated biphenyls) which are neurotoxic, hormone-disrupting chemicals that were banned in the U.S. in 1977.

Experts recommended avoiding the highest mercury containing fish such as king mackerel, swordfish, Atlantic halibut, pike, shark, sea bass, tilefish (also known as golden snapper) and canned white albacore tuna.

At the time of this writing, healthy or low-mercury fish include: Arctic char, crawfish, Pacific flounder, herring, king crab, sand dabs, scallops, Pacific sole, tilapia, wild Alaska and Pacific salmon, Pacific halibut, striped bass and sturgeon. Check fish safety websites before purchasing fresh fish since the recommendations change. An excellent website to check for fish safety and mercury levels is the Monterey Bay Aquarium's Seafood Watch.

Canned tuna is extremely over processed in this country, which makes it devoid of omega-3 fatty acids. However, it is a good source of protein. White tuna in water contains large amounts of mercury, so it is recommended that you purchase light tuna in water since it contains about a third less mercury than white. Oil-packed tuna is usually packed in an omega-6 fat, so it is best to purchase tuna packed in water.

Recommendations for fish during pregnancy are 12 ounces of cooked fish per week and only six ounces of tuna, preferably light tuna in water. In addition, avoiding raw fish is recommended.

· ·

In the preceding pages, we have looked at how carbohydrate, protein and fat work in the diet. Now, let's talk about how to combine them for balanced meals that will help you achieve optimal blood glucose levels.

Since breakfast sets the blood glucose tone for the entire day, it is *the* most important meal. Having protein and keeping your carbohydrate intake low at breakfast is essential since your body is most insulin resistant when you first wake up.

Suggested Plan:

- 2-4 protein servings (14-28 g)
- 1-2 carbohydrate servings (15-30 g)
- 1 fat serving (5 g)

Option 1:
- 2 scrambled eggs with ¼ cup of grated hard cheese and ¼ avocado
- 1 cup of fresh fruit or 1 medium piece of fruit *

Option 2:
- ½ cup of cottage cheese mixed with ½ cup of ricotta cheese*
- ½ cup of fresh fruit*
- 2 tbsp. of raw or dry roasted nuts or seeds of your choice

Option 3:
- ¾ cup of plain low-fat yogurt mixed with a ¼ cup of cottage cheese*
- ½ cup of fresh fruit or frozen berries*
- 2 tbsp. of raw or dry roasted nuts or seeds

*Checking your glucose readings within 1-2 hours after the first bite of food will determine if you can tolerate fruit or dairy products at breakfast.

Breakfast Examples

Lunch/Dinner:

- 3-6 protein servings (21-42 g)
- 2-3 carbohydrate servings (30-45 g)
- 2 fat servings (10 g)

Option 1:

- 3-6 ounces of lean meat, chicken/turkey or fish (or other lean protein)
- Non-starchy vegetables and/or salad as desired
- ½-1 cup of whole grains and/or fresh fruit

Option 2:

- 3-6 ounces of lean hamburger or turkey/chicken burger without the bun
- Side salad with vegetables and avocado and/or a side of fruit
- Olive oil and vinegar on the side

Option 3:

- 1-1½ cups of chicken salad, tuna salad, or egg salad
- Piece of medium fresh fruit

Option 4:

- Mixed green salad with vegetables of choice, 3-6 ounces of lean protein, ½ -1 ounce of cheese, ⅓ of a medium avocado, 1-2 tbsp. of nuts, and olive oil and vinegar for dressing (1-2 tbsp.)

Vegetarian options:

Option 1:

- 1 cup of cottage cheese
- ½ avocado
- ½ medium tomato, quartered
- ½ cup garbanzo beans

Option 2:

- Grilled Portobello mushroom with olive oil
- ½ cup beans or lentils
- ½-1 cup of Greek-style yogurt

Option 3:

- 2-3 eggs
- 1-2 cups of grilled vegetables of choice
- ½ cup of brown rice or quinoa

Snack:

- 1-2 protein servings (7-14 g)
- 1-2 carbohydrate servings (15-30 g)

- 1 ounce of nuts (about 15-20) or seeds (varies) with a medium-sized fruit
- 1-2 slices or ounces of cheese with medium fruit
- 1-2 tablespoons of natural nut butter and a piece of fruit or celery
- Hummus or guacamole (¼ cup) and cut up raw vegetables

Wendy's Story

From Fearful to Empowered

I was pregnant with twins when I was diagnosed with gestational diabetes at 28 weeks. It was just after my birthday, and I was convinced it was because I ate chocolate cream pie. Did I say a slice a pie? I meant the whole pie! I had been pregnant twice before and never tested positive for GDM. I demanded the doctor let me repeat the test, and he informed me that I had to do the three-hour glucose test. I was certain I would pass it this time. When I got the results a week later and found out I failed the test, I was concerned. After searching the Internet, I was terrified my babies were going to come out with scrawny bodies and huge heads.

I continued to gather information and spoke with many people, but I just kept getting confused by all the material. I wasn't sure if I was supposed to count carbohydrate grams or count carb exchanges or what I was suppose to count. I was confused on what foods I could and couldn't eat. Most of all, I was afraid my twins' health was in jeopardy and that they may have diabetes someday. The only thing I did know was that I was not going on insulin. I just had to figure out how to avoid it.

"I was afraid my twins' health was in jeopardy and that they may have diabetes someday."

Finally, I found Susan's website and called her for advice. I had so many questions. First, Susan explained what was happening to my body and the effects it could be having on my twins. She explained how to check my blood sugar and when to check it throughout the day. We discussed what I was eating and some of the modifications I needed to make immediately. Because I live on the other side of the country, she was able to set up a

meal plan for me via email and sessions on the phone.
I followed Susan's meal plan and was able to keep my blood
sugar level under control for the rest of my pregnancy. I never
had to go on insulin.

A year later, I still follow Susan's meal plan. I no longer have
problems with my blood sugars. I have continued to stay on the
meal plan because I feel better overall. I have more energy and
can sleep through the whole night without waking up hungry. I
believe her plan has helped me to drop my baby weight faster
than my previous pregnancies, too. Thank you, Susan, for all of
your guidance and patience! We both know I would have been
put on insulin if I continued down the path I was going.

Wendy's Advice:

- Good information can be found on the
  Internet, but some is scary and inaccurate.
  Be sure to check any advice you read with
  your doctor, dietitian or other healthcare
  professional before you act on it.

- Create your meal plan and stick with it.

2 Checking Your Blood Glucose Levels

One of the best and most efficient ways to know exactly what is going on inside your body is to check your blood glucose levels. With the right equipment, you can do this at home, and it is a powerful tool for gathering information. Trading off a little inconvenience, you'll be able to find out what impact different food combinations are having on your unique physiology.

The times to check your glucose levels are first thing in the morning and then 1-2 hours after the first bite of each meal.

Test your blood glucose:

- Within a few minutes of waking before you eat anything (fasting level)
- 1-2 hours after the first bite of breakfast, lunch and dinner

Testing your fasting blood glucose within a few minutes of waking is important since moving around and starting your day can raise your glucose levels slightly, which skews the ability to get an accurate reading.

The fasting level should be less than 90 mg/dl. If it is higher than 90, your diet and/or exercise level need an adjustment. A poor night's sleep or an illness can also raise your blood glucose levels.

Normal blood glucose values are 70-130 mg/dl. Glucose levels after meals are known as postprandial levels and should be less than 130 mg/dl. However, during the third trimester, blood glucose levels can drop as low as 50 mg/dl, which is considered normal in pregnancy.

Blood Glucose Goals:

Fasting	Less than 90 mg/dl
1-2 hours after first bite of meal	Less than 130 mg/dl

Glucometers

You will need to buy a glucometer to check your blood glucose levels. There are many different types, but they all do essentially the same thing. Ask your healthcare professional or pharmacist which one he or she recommends for ease and cost. In addition to purchasing a glucometer, you will need:

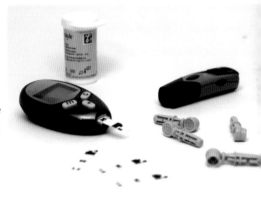

- Lancets (the needle that is inserted into the lancing device which draws your blood)
- Test strips

Some glucometers come with a few of these items for starters, but most do not. Glucometers and lancets are reasonably priced, but test strips are more costly. Many times your healthcare provider can provide you with a complimentary glucometer.

When you get ready to check, wash your hands with warm water and soap and dry with a paper or cloth towel. You can use the needle for the lancet up to three times or for 24 hours (**and only on you**). You may be able to use a needle more than three times, but the lancets will become dull and you will have greater difficulty in getting enough blood for testing.

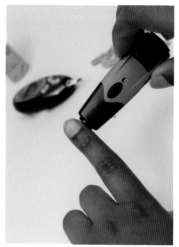

IMPORTANT: If you are sharing a glucometer with someone else, you will need to change the lancet each time.

Prick on the sides of your fingers and alternate both the sides and the fingers. Pricking the finger tips is not only more painful, but increases the possibility of infection since we use our fingertips constantly.

Important!

Blood Glucose Levels and Your Baby

If your blood glucose levels are in the 140 range, your baby will not be harmed, but he or she may be larger at delivery. If your values are in the 160-180 range, it puts stress on your baby's pancreas as it is developing. Insulin does not cross the placenta but glucose does.

Having a chronically high glucose level during pregnancy wears out the pancreas of the baby before it is born, which predisposes your child to adult diabetes later in life.

Factors Affecting Glucose Levels

Blood glucose levels are a curious thing and can be influenced by anything from food to your activity level to the weather. (Really!)

Food

Keeping your diet in balance is the most important thing in regulating your glucose levels. Including protein at meals and snacks is essential since it is proven to lower the blood glucose spike and resulting drop. Carbohydrate in the allowed amounts is also critical. Your body cannot handle a large amount of carbohydrate at one sitting due to the changes in hormones caused by pregnancy. In addition, regular meals are essential to keeping blood glucose values normal. *Make sure you eat every 2-4 hours depending on your values and hunger levels*.

To keep your blood glucose in control:

- Start with a protein source (refer to page 25) such as meat, chicken, fish, cottage cheese, yogurt, etc.

- Balance it with a healthy source of carbohydrate (in the recommended amount), such as a fruit, vegetable, or small amount of non-processed starch (brown rice, quinoa, yam)

- Round out your meal with a healthy fat such as nuts/seeds, avocado or olive oil

Exercise

It is only recently in Western culture that we have begun to look at pregnancy as a delicate state. When you look at civilizations since the beginning of time, there was little change between the activities women did when they were pregnant versus not pregnant. Gestational diabetes is considered a new phenomenon that started in the Western world and is rising due to our food supply, eating habits, and lack of exercise/activity.

Exercise might be the magic pill that wins the blood glucose race, and is equally as important as diet. Raul Artal, MD, an expert in pregnancy and exercise states:

"Pregnant women should walk after each meal to help their insulin work more effectively or walk at least 30 minutes per day. Within 10 days of initiating an exercise program, 60 percent of women with GDM will attain normal blood sugars." [4]

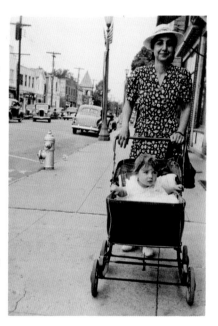

Exercising at least a half hour per day is important and can be divided up in segments. The most important thing is the total time. For women with a high morning blood glucose, a walk after dinner can be very helpful in lowering morning glucose levels.

Other Factors

Other variables that raise blood glucose levels are:

- Weather shifts
- Colds and flu
- Poor sleep
- Stress

Although weather changes are beyond our control, getting your rest is important in controlling your glucose level. Getting proper rest is essential to wake up to a good blood glucose reading. Less sleep raises the blood glucose since it makes the insulin more resistant and less effective.

If someone in your family is sick, try to avoid or limit your contact and frequently wash your hands. Remember to limit touching your face to prevent the spread of germs. If you have a high level of stress, prenatal yoga or meditation can be very helpful. Yoga can re-balance your hormone levels, which will lower your level of insulin resistance hence lowering your blood glucose levels.

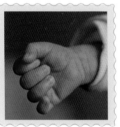

"Children are a handful sometimes,
a heartfull all the time."

- Author unknown

Possible Scenarios and Questions

Why is my blood glucose higher in the morning than before bedtime?

Throughout the day, carbohydrate that is not utilized by the cells of your body or stored as fat gets shuttled to the liver. Overnight, your liver can release the extra carbohydrate into your bloodstream, which will result in a higher morning blood glucose level than when you went to bed. Try the strategies below to assist with keeping your morning glucose levels within normal range.

In addition, keeping a journal of your food and blood glucose readings allows you and your healthcare professional to see patterns and to identify what specific foods raise or lower your blood glucose levels.

A high morning blood glucose

If you're not sick, have had enough rest and still have a morning blood glucose level above 90, here's what can you do to lower your levels:

- Walk daily, especially after dinner or before bed for 10 minutes

- Lower your amount of carbohydrate at dinner to 15-30 grams. Choose salad and a small serving of fruit or some vegetables and a 4-ounce glass of milk

- Limit fruit at dinner or stick to a ½ cup serving

- Have a snack of 1-2 ounces/slices of hard cheese at bedtime

- Lower your level of carbohydrate to 15 grams at breakfast. Try to eat 5 grams less than your usual amounts at lunch and dinner

Why do I feel worse now that my blood glucose levels are becoming normal?

If your blood glucoses levels have been elevated for a few weeks, your body starts to sense these higher levels as "normal" even though they are elevated. The transition of the blood glucose going down from a high to a normal range is a change. This change can result in feeling fatigued, sleepy, or moody. Once your blood glucose is normalized (after a week or two) you will feel better, have more energy and gain a better overall sense of well being. Be patient with yourself through this process of transition.

My blood glucose levels are all over the place. I woke up with an 80, had breakfast and now my reading is 220 two hours later. I feel like a yo-yo. Help!

With GDM you can be prone to rapid changes in blood glucose levels. If you consume more carbohydrates than your body can handle, it can result in a high blood glucose. This will be followed by a spike in your insulin levels and a resulting drop. These large fluctuations can affect your energy and mood.

Some protein at each meal with some healthy sources of fat is important for blood glucose stabilization (refer to page 25). Consuming a set amount of carbohydrate (see pages 32-33) is also necessary to maintain a stable blood glucose reading.

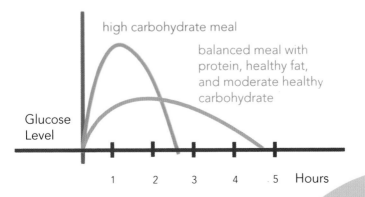

high carbohydrate meal

balanced meal with protein, healthy fat, and moderate healthy carbohydrate

Glucose Level

1   2   3   4   5   Hours

Even healthy sources of carbohydrate that contain more sugar or starch (e.g. fruit, beans/lentils, brown rice, and yams) can trigger spikes in blood glucose levels. Test out different ones to see how your body reacts, since blood glucose shifts in response to food are individual.

I have a lot of carbohydrate cravings – please help! I want to eat the whole cookie jar.

Carbohydrate cravings are common and normal. Remember, the insulin your body makes is more resistant, which contributes to the cravings. Knowing the biology of what is going on helps you know your behavior is not crazy.

Having a healthy source of carbohydrate, like an apple with some sliced hard cheese or natural peanut butter, gives you some sweet and protein to help with satiation. If the cravings are more intense, try 1-2 squares of high-quality dark chocolate (over 70 percent) with 1-2 tbsp. of natural peanut butter. A small amount of dark chocolate will not increase your blood glucose levels if it is limited and eaten with some protein.

Since I've been following the GDM diet I've lost some weight. Is this normal?

In a word – yes. Since your pancreas is working hard to try to normalize your glucose levels, high levels of insulin can cause significant fluid retention, which can increase your weight more than a few pounds.

When you shift your diet to increase the protein and lower the carbohydrate content, your insulin levels calm down, which can result in fluid loss. In fact, your weight may remain flat for 1-2 weeks, which is normal.

In addition, since you are watching your food intake more carefully, a little fat loss can occur. Either way, your physician will monitor the weight of your baby to ensure the safety of your diet and your baby's health.

I'm not sure how to schedule my day to fit in meals, snacks, exercise and testing my glucose values at the right times. Can you give me an example of what is typical?

Scheduling your day with all the necessary things to do and eat is a little challenging at first, but after a few days it will become easier. The following is an example to help you put together a schedule – adjust according to your needs and see pages 32-33 for more meal examples.

7:00 a.m.	Check blood glucose upon waking
7:15 a.m.	Breakfast – 2 eggs scrambled with cheese and veggies, 1 cup of berries and sliced avocado, ½ cup of plain yogurt with 1 tbsp. of ground flax seeds (2 carb servings) * With breakfast take your prenatal vitamin, omega-3s, and vitamin D and other medications as needed.
8:45 a.m.	Check blood glucose level
9:30 a.m.	Morning snack – 1 ounce of almonds (about 20) with a medium fruit (1.5 carb servings)
Noon	Lunch – Tuna salad made with 4 ounces of tuna, 1 tbsp. each of olive oil and vinegar, tomato and lettuce open-faced on 1 slice of whole wheat bread with a medium fruit and carrot slices with ¼ cup hummus (3 carb servings)
1:30 p.m.	Check blood glucose level
3:00 p.m.	Snack – 2 tbsp. natural peanut butter on medium apple or celery (1.5 carb servings)
4:00 p.m.	Take 30-minute walk
6:00 p.m.	Dinner – 4 ounces of chicken breast or steak (or 1 cup of cottage cheese for vegetarian option), 1 cup of grilled veggies, medium yam with 1 teaspoon of organic butter and cinnamon (3 carb servings)
7:30 p.m.	Check blood glucose level
9:30 p.m.	Snack – 2 slices/ounces of hard cheese with ½ apple (½ carb serving)
10:00 p.m.	Bed

Jessica's Story

Taking Back Control

I was six months pregnant when I had found out I had gestational diabetes. I took the second test right before Christmas when my husband and I took our "babymoon" in Maui. Looking back, I should have realized something was off. I was drinking 5-7 glasses of water with every meal, and each time I ate a delicious Hawaiian shaved ice, I ended up washing it down with a gallon of water, which did not seem normal.

When we returned from Hawaii, my midwife left me a message that my sugars were too high, and I needed to call Susan and schedule an appointment immediately. I remember feeling so scared and disappointed in myself. I thought it was all my fault; I should have done things differently and now my baby was at risk.

Susan returned my call that day and I saw her shortly thereafter. She showed me how to take my blood sugar (which was high) and told me everything I could eat. That meant everything else was out. It was a restrictive diet, and I admit I was bummed, but more importantly, I felt in control for the first time, and I knew my baby was going to be okay.

> *"I felt in control for the first time, and I knew my baby was going to be okay."*

Right after my appointment, I bought everything from my glucometer to my supplements and started my new diet. That night my blood sugar was well below where it needed to be. The next week I was cranky and light-headed from the carb and sugar withdrawals, but it got better. I enjoyed cooking many of the recipes from Susan's first book, *A Recipe for Life by the Doctor's Dietitian.*

Throughout the rest of my pregnancy, my blood sugars remained below 100 most of the time. My sugars spiked a few times, but Susan was able to tell me what in my diet had caused this. I learned also what foods to stay away from - like dried fruits.

In the end I gave birth to a very healthy baby girl, born 8 lbs 11 oz, 20 inches. I saw my midwife a week later and found out I was seven pounds lighter than when I first got pregnant, something she said she only sees once every 10 years!

I'm not as strict with my diet now, but there are some foods, like juice and cereal, that I will never go back to eating. This has been a life-changing experience. It is so powerful to be in control of what you put in your body. My baby is thriving, physically, mentally and emotionally, and I do believe that this diet has contributed to her incredible development.

Jessica's Advice:

- Get a glucometer and use it to monitor your blood glucose levels. Looking at the "spikes" will help you learn what foods to stay away from.

- As you change from your regular diet to the GDM diet, you may feel cranky and lightheaded from sugar and carb withdrawls, but hang in there. It does get better!

3 Helpful Hints Along the Way

Supplements

In addition to the correct balance of nutrients, supplements can be very helpful in contributing to and achieving normal blood sugars. This section contains information on some supplements you may want to consider.

Omega-3

Omega-3 fats can reduce the chances of your child being overweight at birth, having a high cholesterol level or experiencing internal inflammation. See the "Fat" section for more information on omega-3 fats (including fish oil as a supplement). Adequate intake of omega-3 fats (ALA, DHA and EPA) through diet and supplements can be essential to normalizing your blood sugars.

Vitamin D

Vitamin D is much more than a vitamin. It functions as a hormone with 37 different tissues requiring its use. [5] Vitamin D is needed for bone metabolism, as well as the development of other systems in the body such as cardiovascular health, neurodevelopment, immunity, insulin secretion and growth in general. [6]

According to researchers from the University of Toronto:

"The period from pre-pregnancy to 24 months of a child's life offers an important developmental window during which vitamin D exposure can have profound effects on human health. Inadequate concentrations of vitamin D during perinatal life can adversely affect bone health, brain development, heart disease, type one diabetes, and cancer. To achieve optimal health at adulthood, it is imperative that pregnant mothers and their newborn babies receive sufficient amounts of vitamin D during critical developmental windows."[7]

Taking extra vitamin D during pregnancy is essential. Have your levels measured twice during your pregnancy – once at the beginning and once during your third trimester to ensure your levels are adequate.

Research shows pregnant women may need at least 4,000-5,000 IU of vitamin D per day both during pregnancy and lactation. Having adequate vitamin D levels helps prevent complications during pregnancy such as preeclampsia and increased levels of insulin resistance leading to high blood glucose levels. [8, 9]

Evidence is also accumulating for the role vitamin D plays in maintaining normal glucose homeostasis. For instance, in both animal and human studies, vitamin D depletion was significantly related to insulin resistance and impaired insulin secretion. Notably, this condition can be reversed by satisfying vitamin D intake. [10]

> **Healthy To-Do:** Have your vitamin D levels checked, but taking a supplement is essential to your health and your baby's health. Most researchers recommend a daily supplement of 4,000-5,000 IU during pregnancy.

Vitamin C

Researchers from the University of Washington examined the levels of vitamin C in the diet of pregnant women. Those who consumed very few fruits and vegetables or less than 70 mg. per day of dietary vitamin C had a nearly four-fold increase in GDM as opposed to those who had higher levels of vitamin C in their diets. [11]

Eating fruits and vegetables on a daily basis can have a huge impact on whether you have GDM or not. Make it a priority to consume at least 1-2 fruits or vegetables high in vitamin C per day such as red peppers, strawberries, oranges and green leafy vegetables. Get a taste for a variety of fruits and vegetables. Mix it up to prevent boredom in your diet and experiment with different spices for flavor and taste.

Fiber

Fiber is an important part of your eating plan. Fiber from fruit, vegetables, salads, nuts/seeds and small servings (about ½ cup) of whole grain carbohydrates such as brown rice or quinoa can lower your blood sugars and reduces the chance of needing insulin.

In addition, it can reduce the chance of your child being overweight at birth by as much as 33 percent. [12]

> **Healthy To-Do:** Increasing fruits and vegetables not only adds nutrients and fiber, but helps your baby's weight be normal and healthy.

Exercise

Statistics show that as soon as women in the Western world become pregnant, they reduce their exercise by 76 percent. This is unfortunate as a simple walk a day reduces GDM by 30-40 percent, and vigorous exercise reduces GDM by at least 55 percent.

Raul Artal, MD, maintains pregnant women need at least 1,400 exercise calories per week to attain normal blood sugars.[4] This number translates to walking at least two miles per day or about 30-40 minutes depending on how fast you walk.

How else can you achieve 1,400 exercise calories per
Since the body likes consistency, it is helpful to do s
each day. Here are a few other examples of ways t
approximately 200 exercise calories per day:

- 30 minutes of low impact aerobics
- 30 minutes of stationary biking or
  using an elliptical machine
- 1 hour of leisurely biking
- 1 hour of a dance class
- 1 hour yoga class

Calories utilized are different depending on how hard you are
working, what your body weight is, the type of equipment you
are using and the exercise class you are taking.

Juice

Although we have been led to believe that juice is healthy, the
body interprets juice the same as it does soda - too much sugar.
Lydia Bazzano, MD, PhD, studied more than 70,000 women
nurses for more than 18 years. Her study showed that women
consuming even one or more cups of juice per day had a 24
percent increased risk of GDM. [13]

Similar studies have shown women drinking juices or sodas have
increased risk of GDM. [13, 14, 15]

> **Healthy To-Do:** Safe beverages during pregnancy are
> water, sparkling waters, iced or hot tea (1-2 cups per day)
> and milk. Ban juices, sodas, sweetened coffee drinks and
> anything containing sugar, fake sweeteners, etc. Your
> body and baby will thank you.

Charting a Healthier Family History

When I received my diagnosis of gestational diabetes at 25 weeks, I was devastated. Even though I have a family history of diabetes, the reality was difficult to accept. I believed that because I had not been eating healthfully enough and exercising more that I had caused myself to get sick. Furthermore, I was angry at my genetics. Ultimately, I was worried that I had already negatively affected my unborn baby's health.

Susan recommended a glucose testing kit and showed me how to check my sugars four times per day. She told me to email her the numbers each night. She gave me meal options and explained my goals for my glucose numbers and also suggested daily exercise to help with insulin resistance. While I was still not thrilled with this new burden, I was beginning to feel a bit more in control of things.

The following months were a bit of a rollercoaster. Most of the time, I managed to test my sugars on time, and with a few exceptions, my numbers stayed under control. There were some instances where I found myself in a panic due to elevated numbers. I would frantically contact Susan, explain what I had eaten, and ask for guidance. She always quickly and calmly responded, explaining the reason for the elevated number and suggesting something to help get me back on track.

I definitely mourned the loss of "fun" foods (like cake at my baby shower) and found myself frustrated when having to turn down even seemingly harmless foods like a glass of milk. In my most difficult moments, I tried to remember that I was giving my baby his first and perhaps one of his most important lessons: how to be healthy. And, most importantly, my baby ended up measuring average (and healthy) on the rest of my ultrasounds.

I know very well that my diagnosis was absolutely a blessing in disguise. Three weeks after starting Susan's eating plan, I discovered I had lost four pounds at my 30-week check-up. For the rest of my pregnancy, I was often told how good and healthy and "glowing" I looked. I gained a total of 11 pounds during my entire pregnancy.

> *"I know very well that my diagnosis was absolutely a blessing in disguise."*

Leslie's Advice:

- Even if you get off track, come back to the basics: organic, whole foods, healthy fats, lean proteins, carbohydrates in the form of fruits and vegetables.

- It's natural to feel upset and angry, but then resolve to make the most of the opportunity to be healthier than you've ever been!

4 Managing Cravings:
Salty and Sweet

It is prevailing wisdom that pregnant women crave certain foods. Whether a factor of physiology or psychology, you may find yourself wanting to reach for something "off the menu" to satisfy a particular urge.

Salty and sweet are two of the strongest cravings I hear from my clients. Salt needs no explanation, but sweet comes into play when women turn to sugar-free products or artificial sweeteners, thinking them acceptable substitutes for sugar, when in fact they do affect blood glucose levels.

In this chapter, I'll share information about both. Some of it may surprise you!

The Skinny on Salt

I'm often asked by my GDM patients if they need to watch their salt intake, and my answer is, "not necessarily." Salt (sodium chloride) is about 40 percent sodium by weight, and a small amount of sodium is essential for proper health and functioning of the body.

More than **70 percent** of the sodium we get in our diet is from processed foods. The remainder comes from salt we use at the table, in cooking, and from sodium that is inherently a part of food.

The average adult gets about **6,000 mg**. of sodium per day. Most health organizations recommend no more than **2,300 mg.** per day. There is no specific guideline for GDM, but staying on the low side is wise.

Since sensitivity to salt has been linked with insulin resistance, having fresh, non-processed foods not only benefits your health, but possibly your blood pressure and glucose levels as well.

In order to lower the amount of sodium in your diet, **avoid or limit:**

- **Processed and prepared foods** – eating a large percentage of foods from a box, can, or package can quickly add up to more sodium than you need. If you are consuming something with a label, look at the sodium level. Stick to foods with less than 200-300 mg. per serving. If you lean toward fresh foods without a label, the natural sodium you receive from these foods will be minimal and adequate.

- **Condiments** – consider the amount in sauces, such as ketchup, barbeque, soy, or specialty sauces. These can pack as much as 2,300 mg. per teaspoon. Broths can also add a fair amount of sodium, so buy the low sodium types. MSG-containing foods have a lot of sodium in them, so it is best to avoid them.

- **Pickled, cured, smoked or preserved foods** – such as pickles, luncheon or cured meats

- **Fast foods, restaurant meals and convenience foods** – just one of these meals can add up to over 2,000 mg. of sodium. Check the nutritional information, if available, and chose options that are lower in sodium.

Enjoy:

- Fresh or ground herbs as alternatives to salt
- Choose low-sodium alternatives such as broth or low-sodium soup
- Reduce the amount of salt in recipes or cut it out completely

The Truth about Sweeteners

At a time when you are actively working to manage your blood sugars, you may be tempted to turn to "sugar free" products. There are a plethora of these on the market aimed at both diabetics and dieters. You'll find pudding, yogurt, diet sodas, iced teas, and the list goes on. These may be marked "free" but they have a real cost when it comes to your long-term health.

Sweet and Low™ (saccharin), NutraSweet™ (aspartame) and Splenda™ (sucralose) are some of the non-nutritive or artificial sweetener brand names you may know. There's also Acesulfamine K and Neotame, the newest one to hit the market. These products all range from half as sweet as sugar to 8,000 times sweeter than sugar, with the average being 200-500 times sweeter than sugar.

Many diet programs and healthcare professionals highly advocate the use of these sweeteners and foods containing them to decrease the amount of sugar and calories a person takes in and to lower blood sugar levels. What is interesting, however, is that the longer these sweeteners have been around, the more obese our nation has become.

Here's the reason why: when you consume alternative sweeteners, you are trying to fool your body. But you can't! The body knows that what you are giving it is fake, so instead of being satisfied, it continues to give the signal that it wants to consume something sweet. This compounds the cravings that someone with or without diabetes might experience naturally.

Research Reveals Risks

In 2008, a study published in the *Journal of Circulation* followed the health status of 9,500 men and women, ages 45-64, over a period of nine years.[16] The researchers found that the typical Western diet increased levels of metabolic syndrome or insulin resistance. The most surprising results of the study linked drinking a diet soda each day to a 34 percent increased risk for metabolic syndrome (insulin resistance) compared to those who drank none.

Another study in *Behavioral Science* in February 2008 at Purdue University compared rats that ate regular feed plus yogurt sweetened with saccharin to rats that ate regular feed plus yogurt sweetened with regular sugar.[17]

The rats who ate the feed plus the saccharin-sweetened yogurt took in 20 percent more calories than with regular sugar (the control group) and they gained body fat. Researchers have theorized that taking in large amounts of non-nutritive sweeteners over time conditions the body not to associate sweetness with calories, which can then disrupt the body's ability to assess caloric intake accurately and lead to overeating.

In countries where more fresh food is consumed than processed food, obesity is not as prevalent. The epidemic of obesity in the U.S. is due, at least in part, to the heavy consumption of products that create the illusion that you can eat more and more of them without gaining weight. The human body was made to process real foods that are fresh and whole, not manufactured processed foods.

Sugar Alcohols

So, what about sugar alcohols like *maltitol* or *xylitol*? Are they viable alternatives? Sugar alcohols are in many foods including mints and chewing gums so be sure to check labels for everything you eat or chew.

The premise behind these carbohydrates from fiber or alcohol sugar is that since they are not digested like regular sources of carbohydrate, they have minimal effects on blood sugar levels. Maltitol is one of the primary alcohol sugars found in foods, and despite the premise, it **does** increase blood sugar. Carbohydrates are equal to 4 calories per gram and maltitol is approximately 3 calories per gram. Fiber does add bulk to food, but to think it **does not** add any calories or impact blood sugars has not been proven by research.

In order to fool consumers into thinking products are low-carb, the food industry made up the term "net carbs." What does this mean? To arrive at a net carb number, food manufacturers take carbohydrates coming from fiber or from alcohol sugars like maltitol and subtract them from the total amount of carbohydrates. This is misleading since it has you believe you are consuming fewer carbohydrates than you actually are.

In addition, all alcohol sugars contain laxative side effects and can contribute to gas, bloating and diarrhea – not a good trade-off for a little sweetness in my opinion!

Agave

Agave, which comes from the cactus and has been used to make tequila, hit the market a few years ago. You can find agave as a sweetener in most products found in health food stores…but is it really a health product? And an interesting fact is that agave is actually more detrimental than high fructose corn syrup.

Using high fructose corn syrup is a cheap way to sweeten foods. It was developed to help food companies cut costs. Whereas real sugar is 50 percent glucose and 50 percent fructose, high fructose corn syrup is approximately 40-45 percent glucose and 55-60 fructose, and not the natural kind like in fruit. When you consume a large percentage of this type of fructose, it gets processed directly by your liver, which not only increases your triglyceride levels, but causes fatty liver, increased hunger levels and a plethora of other health issues you would rather avoid. High levels of fructose make your brain deaf to leptin, the hormone responsible for making you feel full.

With agave, the percentages are altered more significantly - the syrup is 85-90 percent fructose and 10-15 percent glucose. The agave plant goes through heavy processing in order to concentrate it into a sweet syrup. Rather than being natural as we've been led to believe, it is actually a processed food, often with few quality controls.

Summing Up

Salt: Use fresh or ground herbs as an alternative to salt; choose low-sodium alternatives (such as low-sodium broth or soup). Reduce the amount of salt in recipes or cut it out completely. If you are eating out, limit high sodium choices and don't be afraid to ask questions about how food is prepared.

Sweeteners: Staying away from sugar-free products keeps your sugar cravings at bay, your blood sugars under control and lessens your risks of long-term health problems. If you need a little sweet, add a small amount (1 teaspoon) of 100% cane sugar or honey. At this time when you are looking to take extra care of yourself and your baby, what can be sweeter than that?

5 Medications:
Glyburide, Metformin and Insulin

Although I strongly advocate diet and exercise as the first line of treatment for GDM, there are instances where medications during pregnancy may be necessary. If your situation warrants taking medication, what types are available and what do they do? There are two categories – oral medication and insulin. In this section, I'll explain what they do, possible side effects, and how you can help them do their job.

Oral Medications

Two types of oral medications are considered safe during pregnancy. Criteria for drugs taken during pregnancy are safety and efficacy.

Glyburide is an older type of diabetes medication known as an oral-hypoglycemic agent. It triggers the pancreas to release more insulin to help with normalizing blood sugars. Glyburide has not been shown to be harmful to the baby and is effective in many patients with GDM, but not all.

Possible Side Effects: If you are prescribed glyburide, one precaution to be aware of is developing hypoglycemia or low blood sugar.

Healthy To-Do:

Carrying a snack with you, such as an ounce of nuts and a medium apple, is essential in case of hypoglycemia.

Metformin is another type of medication used in diabetes for the last 15 or so years. Metformin helps lower the blood sugar by lowering the amount of glucose produced by the liver, increasing your body's response to its own insulin, and lowering the amount of glucose absorbed from the food you eat. The level of insulin resistance in your body is decreased, which can keep your glucose levels under control.

Metformin **does** cross the placenta. However, Janet Rowan, MD, an expert in GDM states, "Metformin crossing the placenta can be advantageous since it alters the nutrient handling of glucose and cholesterol. This, in turn, can be advantageous for the baby for the future since it can lower the level of future insulin resistance or risk of metabolic syndrome later in life." [18]

Dr. Rowan says she has observed less neonatal hypoglycemia (low blood sugar) in women treated with metformin than glyburide or insulin. She feels this medication improves insulin sensitivity and prevalence of fat deposits in both the mother and fetus. Her 2008 study in the *New England Journal of Medicine* concluded that in women with GDM, metformin was not associated with increased perinatal complications as compared to insulin, with women preferring metformin to insulin treatment. [19]

Possible Side Effects: Metformin can initially cause gas, bloating and/or diarrhea. If started slowly, these side effects can be minimized, are usually temporary, and subside within a week or two. Hypoglycemia is also possible but not common with metformin.

Healthy To-Do:

Take metformin with a meal, preferably with the first few bites. Depending on how much medication your physician prescribes, metformin can be taken 1-3 times a day with meals.

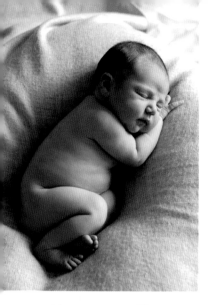

Insulin

Until recently, most women with GDM were not given the choice, but were put immediately on insulin. Oded Langer, MD, a specialist in GDM, states that glyburide and metformin are as effective as insulin. He feels they are all comparable for treatment of GDM depending on the mother and her circumstances. [20]

There are many kinds of insulin, but only a few approved for use with pregnancy. The two categories of insulin are known as *short-* and *long-term insulin*. Short-term insulin is a shot taken before a meal to lower the blood glucose response to what is eaten. Long-term insulin is a shot taken usually once or twice a day to cover blood glucose needs at all other times. It tries to mimic a normal pancreas.

The short-term insulins used are called Lispro, Aspart and regular. [21] The long-term insulin is called NPH. If you are put on insulin, your physician will set up a plan for taking it. This should explain which type, how much and when to take it. It will all depend on your blood glucose levels, your weight, age, and how far along you are in your pregnancy.

Tips for Taking Insulin

Coordinating the types of insulin you are on with meals is a little tricky at first. Figuring out how much insulin to take to match your meals takes some practice. Being in touch with your health-care professional is important to your success.

Regular testing of your glucose levels helps you know exactly how much insulin you need in coordination with the food you eat. Keeping close documentation of the food you eat in coordination with your glucose levels and insulin dosages helps your healthcare provide give clear input for your care. Sometimes it is tempting to give yourself more insulin if your blood sugars don't come down to normal levels. It can take a few hours for insulin to work effectively, so give it time before giving yourself another shot.

Also remember that as the placenta grows, you can become more insulin resistant due to the hormones the placenta makes that block the action of insulin. Therefore, you may need more insulin as you get closer to your delivery date.

Possible Side Effects: Hypoglycemia is a common side effect of giving yourself too much insulin for the meal you are eating, but with practice, you will be able to match your insulin needs with your meals.

Symptoms of hypoglycemia include nausea, sweating or cold clammy skin, anxiety or nervousness, rapid heartbeat or even a mood change or sudden energy drop. If you are taking insulin, regular testing of your glucose levels throughout the day is essential to preventing hypoglycemia.

If you feel the above symptoms and your blood glucose is low (normally less than 70) the treatment is the 15/15 Rule: Immediately eat or drink 15 grams of carbohydrate and retest your glucose levels in 15 minutes. If still low, take another 15 grams of carbohydrate. One of the best treatments for hypoglycemia is 1 cup of whole milk, which contains 15 grams of carbohydrate along with protein and fat to stabilize your glucose levels and prevent another episode of hypoglycemia.

15/15 Rule for Hypoglycemia:

- Eat or drink 15 grams of carbohydrate
- Retest your glucose in 15 minutes and if still low have another 15 grams of carbohydrate

Andie's Story

No-Meds Management

I was diagnosed with unidentified infertility when I was 40. I pursued various fertility treatments, but was told a year later I would not be able to conceive. However, just before my 43rd birthday I found out I was pregnant; I had not used any medications or treatments in over a year. I gave birth to a healthy son at 42 weeks. My second pregnancy was achieved with the use of fertility treatments. At age 47, I delivered a healthy baby girl.

I was diagnosed with gestational diabetes at the beginning of the last trimester of my second pregnancy during a regular OB check up. I was told to contact a registered dietitian and meet back with my OB the following week.

My physician had given me two referrals. One dietitian said she could meet with me in the next 2-3 weeks. Susan was my next call, and she said she could meet with me the following day. During our appointment, Susan told me what foods I could and could not have. She talked to me about the role food, exercise, stress and even colds could play in affecting my blood sugars. She taught me how to take a blood glucose test and what numbers I would be looking for first thing in the morning and after meals.

I kept a log where I wrote down my fasting, breakfast, lunch and dinner test results. If my numbers were too high, I wrote down what I thought contributed, and Susan and I would discuss later. Sometimes it felt like being a detective, trying to determine how much or how little of a particular type of food would alter my test results.

My OB was pushing to put me on oral meds, but I didn't want that, and lucky for me, Susan was there every step of the way guiding me. She helped me tweak my diet almost daily so I could achieve the numbers acceptable to my OB.

> "My OB was pushing to put me on oral meds, but I didn't want that."

It was a more restrictive diet than I was used to, and it took me a few weeks to get a real handle on it. Giving up my decaf lattes was especially tough! I was so sensitive to certain foods that my diet primarily consisted of red meat, chicken, eggs, cheese, fruits and vegetables. Toward the end of my pregnancy I developed ketones. I was able to manage this by adding back daily mini decaf lattes and a little more fruit.

Being diagnosed with GDM was definitely a challenge for me, but I have a beautiful daughter and no lasting effects. I also have the knowledge and experience that I can survive a restricted diet.

Andie's Advice:

- Be your own detective: keep a log for test results -- fasting, breakfast, lunch and dinner

- If your numbers are high, write down what you think contributed and tweak your diet accordingly

6 Closing Thoughts

If you have finished reading this book, it means you are motivated to help your child's future. After your child is born, he or she needs a healthy, vibrant parent to guide them throughout their lives. Managing your lifestyle for maximum health will not only help you as a parent, but models behavior that will shape your child's future health and happiness.

While changing your eating habits isn't easy, a diagnosis of GDM is an early warning sign, and I encourage my clients to see it as a blessing. Women with GDM have a very high likelihood of becoming a type two or adult onset diabetic within 10 years. It is a sign that you need to change your diet or your lifestyle. In doing so, you will have the power to control whether diabetes is in your future.

You may have started this book feeling anxious, but I hope that in reading through it, you have found advice, encouragement and some actions you can take that will be empowering. I also recognize that you may still have some worries – both about this pregnancy and any future pregnancies.

You may be wondering what happens to you or your baby if you can't control your GDM with diet alone. Research shows that women with GDM who are managed well medically during their pregnancies have the same results as women without GDM. If your GDM cannot be managed with diet and lifestyle, there are options available for oral medications and insulin (see the Medications chapter).

It is true that with each pregnancy the chance of GDM increases. Following the healthy diet you adopted during your pregnancy can lower your risk of future GDM. Start preparing for your next pregnancy by achieving a healthy weight and getting regular exercise. Healthy lifestyle behaviors will put you in a positive position at the starting line of your next pregnancy. The changes you make now will have lasting results.

Best wishes and good health for your parenting journey.

Susan B. Dopart, MS, RD, CDE

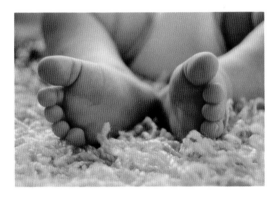

Blood Glucose/Food Journal

	Fasting	Breakfast		Lunch		Dinner		Food/Exercise Comments
			1-2 hrs Post		1-2 hrs Post		1-2 hrs Post	
Mon								
Tues								
Wed								
Thurs								
Fri								
Sat								
Sun								

How can you maximize this chart?

Fasting – the fasting blood glucose level is the one you check within a few minutes of waking. The goal is to have this number below 90 mg/dl. Many times this number is affected by the previous day's eating and/or exercise/activity levels.

Postprandial – this number is one you check within 1-2 hours after your first bite of food. Ask your physician or healthcare practitioner which level is preferred. The goal for this value is below 130 mg/dl. This number can show you what foods make your glucose values normal or elevated.

Glossary

Beta cells – a type of cell located in the pancreas that produces insulin.

Epigenetics – the environmental influence on genes beyond what is encoded in the DNA. As an example, a mother has the ability to change what happens to her child in the womb by lifestyle factors such as diet and exercise.

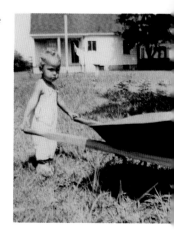

Glyburide – an oral medication used in diabetes that triggers the pancreas to release more insulin to assist with normalizing blood glucose levels.

Glucometer – a monitor used for testing the blood glucose level.

Hyperglycemia – the condition of having a blood glucose level above normal range (more than 130 mg/dl).

Hypoglycemia – the condition of having a blood glucose value below normal range (normally less than 70 in type I and II diabetes, but less than 50 in GDM).

Insulin – a hormone produced by the beta cells in the pancreas that allows glucose to enter the cells for energy. With GDM, it may be necessary to take insulin shots to normalize blood glucose values.

Insulin resistance – a condition that occurs when the body doesn't respond normally to the insulin the pancreas is producing. As a result, it is harder for glucose to enter the cells.

Ketones – substances that are produced when there is insufficient insulin to allow glucose to enter the cells of the body. Instead of using food for energy, fat and muscle tissue are used.

Lancet – a device used to prick the finger to obtain a drop of blood to use on a test strip with a glucometer.

Metformin – an oral medication which assists in lowering blood glucose by lowering the amount of glucose produced by the liver, increasing the body's response to its own insulin, and lowering the amount of glucose absorbed from food.

Omega 3 fats – three types of essential fats known as ALA, DHA and EPA, which lower inflammation in the body and assist in providing important nutrients for the cells in the body and brain. DHA is particularly important for development of the brain in utero.

Preeclampsia – a condition marked by high blood pressure accompanied with a high level of protein in the urine. Women with preeclampsia often have swelling in the feet, legs and hands.

Pancreas – part of the body that serves both as an endocrine gland that produces hormones (including insulin), and a digestive organ that produces enzymes necessary for digestion of food.

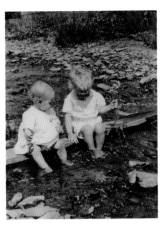

Test strips – disposable strips the glucometer reads and uses to calculate the blood glucose values.

Triglycerides – the storage form of fat in the blood; associated with carbohydrate sensitivity and insulin resistance.

Vitamin D – a hormone that regulates multiple functions in the body and in utero, including bone health, brain development, immunity and insulin resistance.

References

1. Menato, G., et. al. (2008). "Current management of gestational diabetes mellitus." Expert Review of Obstetrics & Gynecology. 3(1):73-91.

2. Hill, D. (April 8, 2010). "Current strategies to manipulate beta cell mass." Presented at the Gestational Diabetes Mellitus International Conference II.

3. Desoye, G. (April 8, 2010). "Placental lipid handling in diabetes." Presented at the Gestational Diabetes Mellitus International Conference II.

4. Artal, R. (April 10, 2010). "Physical activity and GDM." Presented at the Gestational Diabetes Mellitus International Conference II.

5. EcElduff, A. (April 10, 2010). "Micronutrient intake and GDM." Presented at the Gestational Diabetes Mellitus International Conference II.

6. Williams, M. (April 9, 2010). "Early predictors of GDM." Presented at the Gestational Diabetes Mellitus International Conference II.

7. Kaludjerovic, J. and Vieth, R. (Nov/Dec 2010). "Relationship between vitamin D perinatal development and health." Journal of Midwifery & Women's Health. 55(6):550-60.

8. Baker, AM. (August 18, 2010). "A nested case-control study of midgestation vitamin D deficiency and risk of severe preeclampsia." Journal of Clinical Endocrinology and Metabolism. Doi:10.1210/jc.2010-0996.

9. Wagner CL et al. (2010). "Vitamin D supplementation during pregnancy part 2 NICHD/CTSA randomized clinical trial (RCT): outcomes." PAS 2010; Abstract 1665.6.

10. Zhang, C. et al. (November 2008). "Maternal plasma 25-hydroxyvitamin D concentrations and the risk for gestational diabetes." Plos One. 3(11):e3753.

11. Zhang, C. et. al. (Jul., 2002). "Vitamin C and the risk of pre-eclampsia: results from dietary questionnaire and plasma assay." Epidemiology. 13(4): 409-416.

12. Moses, R. (April 10, 2010). "Macronutrient intake and GDM." Presented at the Gestational Diabetes Mellitus International Conference II.

13. Bazzano, LA. et. al. (July 2008). "Intake of fruit, vegetables, and fruit juices and risk of diabetes in women." Diabetes Care. 31(7): 1311-1317.

14. Chen, L. et. al. (December 2009). "Prospective study of pre-gravid sugar-sweetened beverage consumption and the risk of gestational diabetes mellitus." Diabetes Care 32(12): 2236-2241.

15. Hedderson, M. (April 9, 2010). "Pre-gravid predictors of GDM." Presented at the Gestational Diabetes Mellitus International Conference II.

16. Lutsey, PL, et. al. (February 12, 2008). "Dietary intake and the development of metabolic syndrome: the atherosclerosis risk in communities study." Circulation. 117(6):754-61.

17. Swithers, SE, and Davidson, TL. (2008). "A role for sweet taste: calorie predictive relations in energy regulation in rats." Behavioral Neuroscience. Vol. 122(1):161-173.

18. Rowan, J. (April 10, 2010). "Metformin treatment and GDM." Presented at the Gestational Diabetes Mellitus International Conference II.

19. Rowan, J. et.al. (2008). "Metformin versus insulin for the treatment of gestational diabetes." New England Journal of Medicine. 358(19): 2003-2015.

20. Langer, O. (April 10, 2010). "Glyburide treatment and GDM." Presented at the Gestational Diabetes Mellitus International Conference II.

21. Trujillo, A. (2007). "Insulin analogs and pregnancy." Diabetes Spectrum. 20(2):94-101.

Index

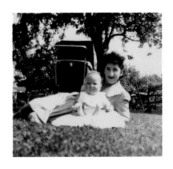

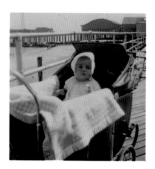

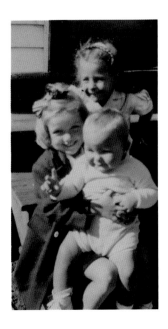

About Susan

Susan B. Dopart, MS, RD, CDE, is a nutrition and fitness consultant who has been in private practice for more than 20 years. Susan specializes in child and adult medical nutrition-related issues associated with insulin resistance, diabetes and endocrinology, pregnancy, infertility, PCOS and exercise. Before establishing her own practice, Susan worked at UCLA as both a medical and kidney dietitian.

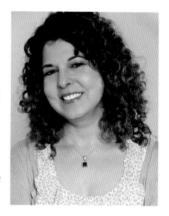

As a consultant, Susan has worked for UCLA Medical Center, UCLA Extension, the Beverly Hills Country Club, Sebastian International and Procter & Gamble. She has written for and contributed to many national and international publications and online websites including, *The Huffington Post, SELF Magazine, UCLA Medicine, Sports and Cardiovascular Nutritionists (SCAN), Best Life, Men's Health, Message Magazine, Diabetes Health and Diabetes Forecast.*

After receiving her bachelor of science degree in nutrition and clinical dietetics from UC Berkeley, Susan earned a master of science degree in exercise physiology and sports medicine from California State University, Hayward. She is a certified diabetes educator (CDE) and a member of the International Motivational

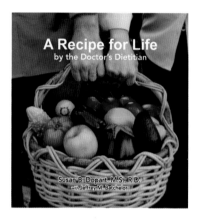

Interviewing Network of Trainers, which practices a collaborative, person-centered form of behavioral change.

Susan is the author of *A Recipe for Life by the Doctor's Dietitian* – a nutrition guidebook, resource, and teaching tool with cutting-edge nutrition information. Her mission and passion are helping her clients find lifestyle solutions for optimal health and well-being. Connect with her online at **www.susandopart.com**.